Visiting People with
DEMENTIA

GW00600979

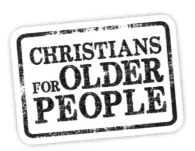

Visiting People with
DEMENTIA

Principles drawn from experience

Janet Jacob

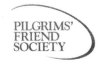

PILGRIMS'
FRIEND
SOCIETY

Visiting People with Dementia

Practical advice drawn from real life experience, and spiritual support.

Copyright July 2014 The Pilgrims' Friend Society.

A catalogue record for this publication is available from the British Library

ISBN: 978-0-9930148-1-9

Designed and typeset by: Pete Barnsley (Creativehoot.com)

Printed and bound by CPI Group (UK) Ltd, Croydon, CR0 4YY

First published in the UK in 2014 by the Pilgrims' Friend Society

175 Tower Bridge Road, London SE1 2AL.
Tel +44 0300 303 1400

Email: info@pilgrimsfriend.org.uk
Website: www.pilgrimsfriend.org.uk

ABOUT THE AUTHOR

Janet Jacob's career has been spent caring for older people. She was a psychogeriatric nurse before becoming a home manager with Pilgrim Homes, now part of the Pilgrims' Friend Society (PFS). Her training and experience proved to be invaluable as more and more older people coming into care were suffering with dementia.

As well as training staff in compassionate and practical dementia care, Janet always found time to comfort and reassure relatives.

Over the last ten years the need for information about dementia has increased as the incidence has surged, and Janet is now part of a team of PFS specialists taking seminars at national events and giving talks in churches and in other organisations.

She receives feedback from participants sometimes years later, telling how what they learnt has changed their lives. The most common response is that now, with a better understanding of what dementia is and how it affects the sufferer, together with the practical advice given they feel encouraged and are better able to cope.

Janet was joint developer of PFS's 'Brain and Soul Boosting for Seniors' sessions; a combination of cognitive and spiritual stimulation for older people, including those with early stage dementia or mild cognitive impairment. She runs the current sessions and has trained churches so they can use the materials within their fellowship and with older people in the wider community.

Janet is also PFS' national exhibitions coordinator, and manages the stand at national events. To the thousands of people who have visited our stands over the years Janet is known as a source of encouragement, as well as information about dementia and other issues of old age.

CONTENTS

'Where shall I go from your Spirit?
Or where shall I flee from your presence?

If I ascend to heaven, you are there!
If I make my bed in Sheol, you are there!

If I take the wings of the morning
and dwell in the uttermost parts of the sea,
even there your hand shall lead me,
and your right hand shall hold me.
If I say, "Surely the darkness shall cover me,
and the light about me be night,"
even the darkness is not dark to you;
the night is bright as the day,
for darkness is as light with you.'

Psalm 139: 7-12

ABOUT DEMENTIA

Dementia is a Latin word that means, literally, apart from, or away from the mind. It is not a description of the disease itself but of the symptoms. There are many different causes of dementia, but in the simplest terms dementia results from physical damage to the brain. Among the main causes are Alzheimer's disease, Lewy Body dementia, vascular infarct (strokes), Pick's disease, Posterior Cortical Atrophy, and Frontotemporal dementia.

The term dementia could become outdated if the updated DSMV, the Diagnostic and Statistical Manual of Mental Disorders (The Psychiatrist's Diagnostic handbook), has its way. The latest edition lists dementia as a neurological disorder and replaces the term 'dementia' with 'major neurocognitive disorder and mild neurocognitive disorder'. However, the authors acknowledge that the disease will probably continue to be called 'dementia', as the name has been widely adopted and is 'snappier' to use.

The symptoms of dementia interfere with an individual's daily activities. These symptoms can include, but are not limited to, forgetting events, names and places, repeating questions, difficulty finding words or putting thoughts in conversation, problems managing money, getting lost in familiar places, trouble doing work or routine tasks, depression, lethargy and apathy, neglecting appearance and personality changes. Although dementia is more common in older people, it is not an inevitable part of ageing.

There is no cure but there are some medications that can help to hold back the progression. Experts acknowledge that the best treatment for people with dementia is the quality of care that they receive. Good care can help to 'hold the person together', and slow the decline.

Dr Jennifer Bute was a General Practitioner until diagnosed with Alzheimer's at the age of 63. She has set up a website sharing information and advice from a personal as well as a professional viewpoint. It is well worth visiting - www.gloriousopportunity.org.

About the Pilgrims' Friend Society

PFS is a Christian charity with roots going back

to August 1807, when the Aged Pilgrims' Friend Society (APFS) was formed by a group of young believers in Islington, London. 1807 was also the year that the Slave Trade Act received its royal assent abolishing the slave trade in the British colonies and making it illegal to carry enslaved people in British ships. Convinced of the value of every individual to God, anti-slave campaigner William Wilberforce, a generous supporter of the charity, became vice president from 1824 until his death in 1835. Other notable Christian friends and benefactors included the Earl of Shaftesbury and the preacher Charles Haddon Spurgeon, who preached sermons on APFS' behalf.

In the early 1800s there was no Welfare State and living conditions in Great Britain were dire. It was the time of the industrial revolution, which brought many people into the cities to earn a living. Children were working in factories and still sweeping chimneys. Elderly people were particularly vulnerable. The founders of APFS report many living in garrets and sleeping on straw, usually possessing only one garment. In those days APFS helped by giving regular pensions, which were always delivered in person, together with spiritual support. The first financial period closed on March 31st, 1808, with a total expenditure of £5 2s. 9d, and by the close of 1830, APFS had paid out in pensions £7,643.16.0d.

The first housing scheme was built in 1835. Today, PFS has sixteen housing and care schemes in different parts of the country, with around 500 people under its wing. A good percentage have dementia, and staff receive specialist training in dementia care. Each scheme also benefits from groups of supporters, known as 'Friends of ... 'who visit and befriend residents and pray for staff. They also receive training in visiting those with dementia. Spiritual support remains a core component of care, particularly its importance for people with dementia.

In addition, PFS helps to support the care of older people in the community by sharing its knowledge and experience with others, at conferences and workshops around the country. More information about this can be found on page 33.

WHY BOTHER VISITING PEOPLE WITH DEMENTIA?

This book is written to help anyone who visits people with dementia, as a friend, relative, or church member. Whether the visit is in the person's home, in a care home, or in hospital, or even in a local park on a summer's day, the principles and practices described here will help.

Dementia is unlike any other disease. It can be very isolating for the sufferer and difficult for visitors, because it affects the normal ability to communicate. Relatives tell us how sad they are when their parents' friends stop visiting. Joan is a pastoral worker who cared for her mother until she reached the stage where she needed to go into a care home. She wrote that her experience of dementia could be summed up in one word: 'loneliness. I watched as friends gave up on her, some people even to the extent of no longer trying to have a conversation, it was as if she wasn't in the room. One person said, 'it's a shame she's lost her personality,' because she was no longer able to reminisce over shared memories. Even health care professionals at medical appointments didn't seem to know how to cope. At times I felt it was me and her against a world that didn't understand or seem to want to.'

Yet Christians are bearers of the most powerful means of communicating imaginable - we are temples of the Holy Spirit, and carry within us the Holy Spirit wherever we go (1 Corinthians 6:9). Jesus was very clear about this, telling His disciples that when He had left them, after the Cross, He would ask the Father to send them the Holy Spirit who would guide and help them, and remind them of all Jesus had told them (John 14:26). *The Holy Spirit is the ultimate communicator.* He tells us things about God, ourselves and about one another. For example, a resident with dementia wouldn't settle one night and the manager asked her friend to pray with her. Imagine the friend's astonishment when the resident prayed for an issue that the friend had kept to herself and that no-one knew about. Another example is the story of Mary visiting her cousin Elizabeth, in Luke's Gospel (Luke 1:41). When Elizabeth heard Mary's greeting, it says that Elizabeth's baby 'leaped in her womb, and Elizabeth was filled with the Holy Spirit' (Luke 1:41).

Deep calls to deep, the Scripture says in Psalm 42. 'Only a call from the depths can provoke a response from the depths, 'Watchman Nee wrote,' nothing shallow can ever touch the depths, nor can anything superficial touch the inward parts. Only the deep will respond to the deep. Anything that does not issue from the depths cannot touch the depths.'

So before we look at practical measures, we can be clear that for Christians there is a means of communication that is beyond all others.

If that sounds super spiritual and a bit ephemeral, consider the experience of Christine Bryden. Christine was a highly placed executive with the Australian Government when she was diagnosed with dementia at the age of 46. She is now aged 62. In the intervening years she has remarried; has become a voice for people with dementia, speaking at national conferences, and has written two books. In an interview with Louise Morse, PFS' media & communications manager in 2014, she said that her neurologist, looking at her brain scans says he does not understand how she is living as fully as she does. Asked what she puts it down to she said, 'The Holy Spirit.'

In a talk at a national conference Christine said:

'As I lose an identity in the world around me,

which is so anxious to define me by what I do and say, rather than who I am,

I can seek an identity by simply being me, a person created in the image of God.

My spiritual self is reflected in the divine and given meaning as a transcendent being ...

As I travel toward the dissolution of myself, my personality, my very 'essence',

my relationship with God needs increasing support from you,

my other in the body of Christ.

Don't abandon me at any stage, for the Holy Spirit connects us. ...

I need you to minister to me, to sing with me, pray with me, to be my memory for me ...

You play a vital role in relating to the soul within me, connecting at this eternal level.

Sing alongside me, touch me, pray with me, and reassure me of your presence,

and through you, of Christ's presence.

I need you to be the Christ-light for me,

to affirm my identity and walk alongside me'.

In another context Christine added,

'I may not be able to affirm you, to remember who you are or whether you visited me. But you have brought Christ to me. If I enjoy your visit, why must I remember it? Why must I remember who you are? Is this just to satisfy your own need for identity? So please allow Christ to work through you. Let me live in the present. If I forget a pleasant memory, it does not mean that it was not important for me.'

Genuine love and concern is what counts when visiting people with dementia, whether in care homes or in their own home. Emotions are heightened as cognitive function fails, and it's love that makes its way through and hearts will respond. Your good 'vibes' will be picked up and dementia sufferers will feel much better as a result of your visit. Your peace will be there also, even though you may not be aware of it. Jesus said, 'Peace I leave with you;

my peace I give you,' (John 14, 27). And that peace can be passed on to another person (as Jesus taught in Luke 10, 5-6).

The time we spend with the person affirms who they are, and helps them to know they are valued and loved. The most precious thing we can do for our brothers and sister in Christ with this illness is to keep affirming them and reminding them of just how precious they are to God.

IMPORTANT THINGS TO DO

a. Preparing beforehand

It's important to prepare to 'just be' with the person with dementia. When we visit someone with dementia we do not always receive the feedback we are used to. The person sometimes doesn't respond. We're not used to this and it makes us feel uncomfortable. Because this vital reciprocity is missing, visitors can go away dissatisfied, feeling that nothing has 'worked' and that the visit was of no use whatsoever. But remember that, as Christine said, you are relating to the soul within, connecting at this eternal level. In *communicating* we look at ways of drawing the person out, but sometimes we have to 'just be'. Sometimes, too, people with dementia are content just to 'be' in your presence, without needing to feel they have to come up with words that may be difficult for them to find. Holding hands can be welcomed by many (ask the caregiver about this in advance) and let your warmth be expressed in your body language and your genuine concern. This will minister, even if you think it isn't doing anything.

Find out as much as possible about the person with dementia. Their caregiver will be able to give you relevant personal information or, if they are in a care home the manager and carers will be able to help. *Knowing* as much as possible about the person is the key.

How does the person like to be addressed? First names may be acceptable, but many older people prefer Mr or Mrs, in the more formal way. Do they need to use a hearing aid, and do they wear spectacles?

Find out, too, about the person's life before they became ill. What was their career? Did they have children? Did they have special hobbies, or did they travel overseas? Many missionaries have lived in foreign countries for most of their working lives. Do they like animals, or music, or photographs? And importantly, is there something they particularly *dislike*?

It may be that some phrases will be especially meaningful and comforting to them and can act as triggers for good or bad. In the World War II Memorial celebrations a few years ago a number of old phrases were resurrected, including, 'Keep Calm and Carry On,' which brought a smile to many older residents.

If the person was an artist, you could take in with you pictures of the sort of art he would appreciate. Missionaries might appreciate photographs of the country in which they worked. People who have been animal lovers might like pictures of dogs, or cats. A former seamstress might like a bag full of different fabrics to go through. Pictures and little videos can be uploaded on to a tablet and shown to the person.

Finding out as much as you can about their interests and their past helps you bring things into the conversation that can bring back memories and feelings. It can also bring a sense of renewed identity: things that they can hook into and which will make them come alive again. You could take in photographs of the area, or the era that they grew up in, or fabrics, or cakes you've baked, or sea shells. Knowing a little about their childhood, war-time experiences, their work, their achievements and talking about these things can help restore a sense of worth, and reawaken zest. And, for the listener, this can actually be quite fascinating. Sometimes school children visit residents in our homes to interview them about their past lives, and they find it captivating. It is usually memory of more recent events that is lost, so focus on the person's earlier life, where the memory can be surprisingly good.

Ask when the best time is to visit; some people are better in the mornings, others in the afternoon or evening. If the person is at home, they may have prior arrangements and if the visit will take place in a residential care home or nursing home they will have their routines.

It might be useful to keep a diary or visitors' book at the person's home, recording what you have done during your visit, and the person's response. This will show other visitors what has been covered and what is working, and will help to plan future visits

b. Communicating

Conversation is fundamental in our everyday lives. Conversing allows us to share, to gather information, and to share what we know. Through speech we express our feelings, hopes and expectations, fears, and beliefs. Someone with dementia who has difficulty with words and speech will try hard to communicate and for them this can be frustrating and physically exhausting. We need to listen carefully to understand what the person is trying to say, and to respond in a way that will promote the person's comfort and confidence. We also need to read the non-verbal communication the person will be displaying such as facial expressions and body language. Some behavioural changes may also be the person's way of trying to communicate by gaining someone's attention.

Always approach a person with dementia from the front, so they can see you coming, and be sure to sit facing them, making good eye contact if possible. Dr Jennifer Bute (the GP we mentioned earlier, who retired early because of dementia), talks about friends and visitors providing the 'rungs on the ladder of her memory' allowing her to continue with conversations. It's the same in ordinary circumstances – how many times have you met someone whose face you remember but not the context in which you know them? So remind the person how you know them and of any connections such as being in the same church or being a neighbour. And remember the power of the Scriptures. Why accentuate the Scriptures? Because they are 'active and living' and have a lasting, beneficial effect, (Hebrews 4:12.)

Gently chat and throw out conversational hooks

that will help stimulate interest and response. If the person is able to converse, allow plenty of time for a response. Other ways to trigger deeper memories are reminders of familiar things like a favourite song, a hymn, a scripture, or a picture of something from the past that will be recognised. Of course, again, you need to know what these triggers are – but you will be rewarded many times over for your effort if you can awaken old feelings through these much loved memories. You will feel you are getting through! And, if you bring a Scripture, bring it in the version that they will have been brought up with (probably the King James Version). Just being there may be enough, and reading Scriptures will bring peace, hope and encouragement – as Christine said, you are bringing a connection with eternity. If you are visiting from the same church, bring news of people and the things that are happening.

Always be open to surprises! In our 'Brain and Soul Boosting' sessions was a gentleman who had largely lost the ability to speak. He found communicating with others in the group very difficult. But one day, as we were thinking about closing in prayer, he suddenly took the initiative and prayed the most appropriate, lovely prayer you could imagine. From then on, until he became too ill to attend, he would close the session in prayer. We find that often when deep resources are tapped the person is able to respond like this.

c. *During your visit*

With dementia we look at the person and not the symptoms. That is why Annie, a Scottish nurse who was diagnosed with Alzheimer's in her forties wrote her life history soon after her diagnosis. She said she wanted to be known for who she is, and not who she may become.

You've done all your preparation; you've found the best time to visit, you've brought mementoes for prompting memory and as 'conversation starters'. You've prayed, and you've prepared your mind for a different sort of visit to those you've most likely experienced beforehand.

This is a list of things to remember and we're using the name 'Bill' to make it real and personal.

- ✓ Approach from the front, and with a smile.

- ✓ If necessary introduce yourself, or remind Bill who you are.

- ✓ If Bill wears a hearing aid or glasses, make sure he has them in place. One of our residents, a little lady called Kathleen, always put her hearing aid in her cardigan pocket. Staff and visitors used to check and remind her to put it on as soon as they arrived.

✓ Always sit close and maintain good eye contact.

✓ Be sensitive to Bill's mood and feelings.

✓ Speak clearly and not too quickly.

✓ Be prepared with an outline of what you may chat about, but be flexible.

✓ Bring news about church events, and people in the fellowship.

✓ Bring news about current events that you know he will be interested in. Discussing a news story about parents sending an invoice to the parents of a child who had not attended their son's birthday party brought an instant response from a mother.

✓ Use visual aids if appropriate, linking them to Bill's life history.

✓ Use topics that their life history will show they are interested in and draw on things they will know, for example events from their childhood, Sunday school songs, familiar hymns and well known Bible stories.

✓ Use hooks, just burbling and throwing out topics that will hopefully engage the person in conversation.

✓ Give the person time to respond- don't be in a hurry.

✓ Don't be afraid of repeating things but do so gently and with patience.

✓ Don't correct Bill if he uses the wrong word in conversation. Sometimes people with dementia do use wrong words because they can't find the right ones.

✓ Don't challenge Bill's version of reality. Research shows that as the condition progresses memories are gradually lost, beginning with the latest. It may be that some people with dementia, at different moments in time are living in a world that is in the past- but it is not an imagined world. They are not being delusional. Their world is very real, but it belongs to the past. They cannot comprehend the present reality because of the brain damage.

✓ If Bill says that his mother is coming to collect him at tea-time, don't tell him that his mother died some years ago. Learn to deflect and divert, but without lying to him. In this instance you could say, 'Ah mothers! They are so precious to us, aren't they! Tell me about your mother.' Or you could tell Bill about your mother.

✓ Keep to one topic at a time and don't change the subject swiftly.

✓ Encourage Bill from the Scriptures, especially if he expresses guilt or fears. Make a note of Hebrews 13:5, 6, 2Timothy 2:19, Psalm 71:18, John 20:30-38, Psalm 103:13-14, Romans 8:28-30 and 34-37.

✓ Speak about Christ and the cross. Talk gently, reminding him of the glories of heaven using Scriptures when you can. John 14: 1-3, Revelation 21: 3-5 and 22: 1-4, Jude 24. There are many more that you probably know well.

✓ Listen to music, especially hymns.

✓ It is always good to end the visit with a brief prayer. Prayer brings calm and a sense of peace as the Holy Spirit ministers.

REMEMBERING THE CAREGIVER

Often the caregiver will be an elderly spouse; others are daughters, sons or friends and neighbours. Their own needs may be neglected, and they can become isolated and lonely because of their responsibilities. From conversations with caregivers we know that they cope better when given the right support and encouragement from their families, friends, churches, and professionals. They need to know their families and friends are still going to be a part of their life; that they will continue to enjoy their company and love and will not allow them to become isolated.

When we are surrounded by empathy and love on all sides we cope better when life gets tough. The Holy Spirit inspired the Psalmist to write, 'As the mountains surround Jerusalem, so the Lord surrounds His people from this time forth and forevermore', Psalm125:2.

Spiritual and emotional support is vital for the caregiver. If they can spare the time and have the energy, pray with them and encourage them with assurances from God's Word. Psalms 36-41 talk of suffering and despair, but also the comfort that David has in knowing God cares for him and understands what he is experiencing. Ask if there are specific prayer requests you can take back to the fellowship.

Practical help is welcome, too. You could also ask if there are any small jobs that someone in the church might be able to do, such as cutting the grass, or helping to fill in forms. Before you do this you will have found volunteers who are happy to give their time in this way.

You may like to take with you a copy of the book, *Worshipping with Dementia*. This contains short, relevant and uplifting devotions that include a Scripture verse, a short passage illustrating the theme, a prayer, and the words of an old hymn. The book was produced with tired caregivers and frail minds in mind. It can be purchased through our website, www.pilgrimsfriend.org.uk, or through Amazon or Christian retailers. But if you purchase through us it helps us a little.

VISITING IN
CARE HOMES

Visiting people in care homes can be a spiritual life-line to them. If it is a secular care home, you may be the only visitor bringing spiritual encouragement and support. It is a very precious opportunity, reflective of Matthew 25:40.

A pastor who preaches regularly in our care homes tells of an experience that radically changed his attitude towards preaching to people with dementia. He said, 'A resident had severe Alzheimer's disease. She possessed a very sweet nature and a lovely smile, but could speak only two or three words. She sat quietly in her chair, mouth open wide and with a completely vacant look. On one occasion, as I gave out my text, her mouth closed, her eyes came alive and were riveted to me the whole time I was preaching. When I concluded, the vacant look returned and her mouth immediately dropped open.

Nothing was clearer to me than that the Holy Spirit had communicated the Word of God to the soul of this elderly saint.'

Most care home staff work very hard, and they are kind to relatives. It is not wise to feel that because you have a captive audience you can freely evangelise care home staff: it is better to be sensitive to the leading of the Holy Spirit.

Find out from staff the best times for visiting. Again, you may find *Worshipping with Dementia* helpful here, too. A retired Vicar, visiting his wife in a local care home said it was invaluable. He also found that other people enjoyed listening, so arranged with staff a time to take a little 'service.' He found others interested in visiting in this way and they formed a team that visited other care homes in the region.

Take time to thank carers for their hard work. See if there are ways you could support the home, for example, by attending special events it may arrange. Ask the manager if there is anything you could do. Not forgetting that prayer is the most powerful support for hard pressed care staff.

EXCERPTS FROM
WORSHIPPING WITH DEMENTIA.

1. A friend to strengthen

Jonathan, Saul's son, arose and went to David into
the woods, and strengthened his hand in God.

1 Samuel 23:16

David was in great difficulty. Chosen by the Lord to
be king, he seems more like a convict in hiding than
a king in waiting. Saul, the current king, is set on
David's destruction. With a large army Saul is hunting
for David and his 600 supporting men. 'Saul looked
for him every day,' reads the Scripture in verse 14.

Think what it must have been like for David, waking
up each morning knowing that Saul might capture him
that day. He would have wondered how the Lord could
fulfil his promise and place him on the throne. Here

he was, having been anointed by Samuel (1 Samuel 16:13), now in danger of being beheaded by Saul.

The woods provided a hiding place for David and his men. Then came a welcome visitor, Jonathan, who loved David and was intent on supporting him. Saul's aim was to kill David. Jonathan, who was Saul's son, had an altogether different aim. He wanted to strengthen David's hand in God.

What a lovely meeting it must have been as Jonathan encouraged and supported David in his time of need and difficulty. Look for some opportunity to meet a godly friend who can strengthen you in your walk with the Lord today. Or perhaps you can be a Jonathan today and strengthen someone in difficulty to continue steadfast in their trust in the Lord.

Prayer

Dear Lord, you directed Jonathan to strengthen David in his hour of need.

Provide a 'Jonathan opportunity' today so that we may all be strengthened in the Lord's good hand.

Amen.

Hymn

Here is love, vast as the ocean,
Loving kindness as the flood,
When the Prince of Life, our Ransom,
Shed for us His precious blood.
Who His love will not remember?
Who can cease to sing His praise?
He can never be forgotten,
Throughout Heav'n's eternal days.

On the mount of crucifixion,
Fountains opened deep and wide;
Through the floodgates of God's mercy
Flowed a vast and gracious tide.
Grace and love, like mighty rivers,
Poured incessant from above,
And Heav'n's peace and perfect justice
Kissed a guilty world in love.

Let me all Thy love accepting,
Love Thee, ever all my days;
Let me seek Thy kingdom only
And my life be to Thy praise;
Thou alone shalt be my glory,

Nothing in the world I see.
Thou hast cleansed and sanctified me,
Thou thyself hast set me free.

In Thy truth Thou dost direct me
By Thy Spirit through Thy Word;
And Thy grace my need is meeting,
As I trust in Thee, my Lord.
Of Thy fullness Thou art pouring
Thy great love and power on me,
Without measure, full and boundless,
Drawing out my heart to Thee.

William Rees, translated by William Edwards, 1900

2. Always with you

He did not take away the pillar of the cloud by day,
nor the pillar of fire by night, from before the people.

Exodus 13:22

Today, whatever your circumstances, you can be
assured of the Lord's abiding presence with you.
The Children of Israel didn't ask for the pillar of
cloud and fire; graciously the Lord gave this physical
sign of His presence leading the people out of
Egypt. He was with them continually, by day and
night. They were never outside of His care, and
neither are you as you trust in Christ.

Look for little signs today of His abiding presence
and love. We may find the Lord's leading in our
lives strange and perplexing. At times we may find
ourselves in a wilderness situation, just like the
Children of Israel. Be encouraged because 'Jehovah
went before them' (verse 21), and He will go ahead
of you today, no matter how difficult it may appear.
The Lord is faithful, protecting and providing for His
pilgrims in this life and in the life to come. In the
Great Commission in Matthew 28:20 we read the
words of Jesus: 'and, behold, I am with you all the
days until the end of the world.'

Prayer

Dear Lord, help us to recognize your presence and love in our lives today.

We thank you for your intimate knowledge of us and your abiding presence with us. We ask forgiveness for our lack of faith and trust.

Amen.

Hymn

I stand amazed in the presence
Of Jesus the Nazarene,
And wonder how He could love me,
A sinner, condemned, unclean.

Refrain:

O how marvellous! O how wonderful!
And my song shall ever be:
O how marvellous! O how wonderful!
Is my Saviour's love for me!

For me it was in the garden He prayed:
'Not My will, but Thine.'
He had no tears for His own griefs,

But sweat drops of blood for mine.

Refrain

> In pity angels beheld Him,
> And came from the world of light
> To comfort Him in the sorrows
> He bore for my soul that night.

Refrain

> He took my sins and my sorrows,
> He made them His very own;
> He bore the burden to Calvary,
> And suffered and died alone.

Refrain

> When with the ransomed in glory
> His face I at last shall see,
> 'Twill be my joy through the ages
> To sing of His love for me.

Refrain

Charles H. H. Gabriel, 1905

HELPING OTHERS CARE FOR OLDER PEOPLE

SUPPORTING AND EQUIPPING OTHERS IN THE COMMUNITY.

Earlier in the book, on page 3, we mention how PFS shares its experience and knowledge to support others' work with older people. With an increasingly ageing population nearly everyone has more older people in their lives, whether they are in their families, their churches, their communities or in their workplaces. On page 33 is a list of some of the topics we are asked to address.

Our speakers include experts in their field, both from PFS and from others in different specialisms. They are all evangelical Christians and they all speak from practical experienceas well as academic knowledge.

We are constantly refining and developing our seminars and workshops. We keep up to date with clinical research on old age and dementia , and we also monitor participants' feedback for issues arising. Typical of feedback comments is one from a daughter who attended one of our conferences on dementia. Five years' later she donated some of her deceased mother's jewellery to auction to aid our funds, and she told us:

> *'What I heard at your seminar I shared with my family. We were caring for our mother at the time, and we'd been considering residential care. But what we learnt enabled us to continue to care for her at home. Thank you from all of us!'*

FINDING OUT MORE ABOUT PFS

We also have a number of publications, including books and booklets that can help.

If you would like to hear more about the issues that affect older people, and how you can help, please visit our website: www.pilgrimsfriend.org.uk, or email info@pilgrimsfriend.org.uk, or telephone 0300 303 1400.

TALKS AND SEMINARS:

1. Making a truly dementia friendly church
2. Dementia – practical and spiritual insights
3. Dementia – the support and help that churches can give
4. Early dementia and the vital circles of support
5. Visiting people with dementia
6. Giving effective support to family caregivers
7. Empowering and engaging older people
8. Caregivers – how to care for yourselves
9. Ministering in care homes
10. Dealing with loneliness
11. How to prepare for a great old age
12. Developing your talents and gifting after retirement
13. Empowering older people
14. Caring for elderly parents and other relatives
15. Building communities, a street at a time
17. Christians and retirement
18. Ensuring a good death
19. Legal issues in old age
20. About death and dying

ORGANISATIONS THAT CAN HELP:

Here is a selection of organisations that are geared up to helping you.

1. **Age UK** (formerly Age Concern and Help The Aged) – the UK's largest charity working with and for older people, with links to local branches.

    Tel: 0800 169 6565;

    website: www.ageuk.org.uk

2. **Alzheimer's Society** – the UK's leading care and research charity for people with dementia and their carers.

    Tel: 0845 300 0336;

    website: www.alzheimers.org.uk

3. **Care Quality Commission** – website shows rating for UK care homes.

    Tel: 03000 616161

    website: www.cqc.org.uk

4. **Carer's Allowance Unit** – part of Department of Work and Pensions, giving advice on the Carer's Allowance, the main state benefit for carers.

    Tel: 0845 608 4321;

    Text Phone: 0845 604 5312

    website: www.direct.gov.uk/en/DI1/Directories/ DG_10011215

5. **Carers' Christian Fellowship** – offers mutual support, sharing and prayer.

   Tel: 023 8028 3270;

   website: www.carerschristianfellowship.org.uk

6. **Carers UK** – offers support with caring for carers.

   Tel: 0808 808 7777;

   website: www.carersuk.org

7. **Counsel and Care** (for older people, their families and carers) – provides personalized and in-depth advice.

   Tel: 0845 300 7585;

   website: www.counselandcare.org.uk

8. **Brunel Care** (incorporating Dementia Care Trust) – offers accommodation, health care, counselling and other assistance, to prolong an independent lifestyle.

   Tel: 0117 914 4200;

   website: www.brunelcare.org.uk

9. **Dementia UK** – offering practical advice and emotional support to people affected by dementia through fully trained Admiral Nurses

   Tel: 020 7874 7200;

   website: www.dementiauk.org

   Admiral Nursing Direct: 0845 257 9406

10. **Dementia Web (formerly DISC)** – an all-age dementia information resource for the UK, providing information about other related services across the UK
Tel: 0845 120 4048;
website: www.dementiaweb.org.uk

11. **Tourism For All** – charity specialising in accessible holiday and respite services for older and disabled people and their carers (helps make tourism welcoming to all).
Tel: 0845 124 9971;
website: www.tourismforall.org.uk

12. **Office of the Public Guardian**
– helps with planning for one's future.
Tel: 0300 456 0300;
website: www.publicguardian.gov.uk

13. **PARCHE** – Pastoral Action in Residential Care Homes for the Elderly; training for church teams.
Tel: 01323 438527;
email: PARCHEenquiries@hotmail.co.uk.
website: www.parche.org.uk

14. **Parish Nursing Ministries UK** – whole person health care through the local church.
Tel: 01788 817904;
website: www.parishnursing.org.uk

15. **The Frontotemporal Dementia Support Group**
    (incorporating Pick's Disease Support Group) – caring
    for people with Frontotemporal dementia, with
    regional links.

    website: www.ftdsg.org

16. **Relatives and Residents Association** – information
    about residential care and help if things go wrong.

    Tel: 020 7359 8136;

    website: www.relres.org

17. **Contented Dementia Trust (formerly SPECAL)**
    – dementia charity providing courses, services and
    advice. Is known best for its themed approach to care.

    email: info@conteddementiatrust.org
    website: www.conteddementiatrust.org

18. **Carers Trust (formerly Princess Royal Trust and
    Crossroads Care)** – works to improve carers' services
    and helps carers make their needs and voices heard.

    Tel: 0844 800 4361
    website: www.carers.org

19. **Independent Age** – advice and information on home
    care, care homes, going into hospital and related issues.

    Tel: 0845 262 1863
    website: www.independentage.org

20. **AT Dementia** – Information on assistive technology for people with dementia.

    Tel: 0116 257 5017

    website: atdementia.org.uk

21. **Guideposts Trust** – provides direct services to people with dementia, their families and carers, to help them make the best choice for care services.

    Tel: 01993 772886;

    website: guidepoststrust.org.uk

22. **Alzheimer's Research UK** – provides information on the different types of dementia, their symptoms and the treatments available to help.

    Tel: 01223 843899

    website: www.alzheimersresearchuk.org

International

23. **Health and Age** – website with contact information for Alzheimer's organisations in various countries.

    website: www.healthandage.com/html/min/adi/page2